No Ordinary Apple

A Story About Eating Mindfully

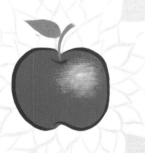

STORY BY **SARA MARLOWE**   ILLUSTRATIONS BY **PHILIP PASCUZZO**

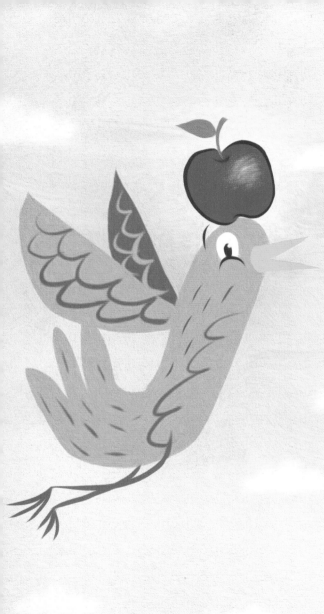

Wisdom Publications
199 Elm Street
Somerville, MA 02144 USA
www.wisdomexperience.org

*To Beckett and Adalyn:
May you always keep
your beginner's mind. —S.M.
To my parents. —P.P.*

Library of Congress Cataloging-in-Publication Data
Marlowe, Sara (Sara Gwynn), 1973–
  No ordinary apple : a story about eating mindfully / story by Sara Marlowe ; illustrations by Philip Pascuzzo.
    p. cm.
  Summary: Elliot stays with his neighbor, Carmen, after school every day and one afternoon she offers an apple as a snack, guiding him to experience it in a new way that makes it "the most appley apple ever."
  ISBN 1-61429-076-8 (cloth : alk. paper)
  [1. Apples—Fiction. 2. Awareness—Fiction.] I. Pascuzzo, Philip, ill. II. Title.
  PZ7.M3455No 2013
  [E]—dc23

                        2012030217

ISBN 978-1-61429-076-6; eBook ISBN 978-1-61429-095-7

25 24 23 22   5 4 3 2

Cover and interior design by Philip Pascuzzo. Set in Futura Bold 13/22.

Wisdom Publications' books are printed on acid-free paper and meet the guidelines for permanence and durability of the Production Guidelines for Book Longevity of the Council on Library Resources.

Printed in Thailand.

SARA MARLOWE is a clinical social worker, mindful self-compassion teacher, singer-songwriter, and foodie. She lives in Toronto with her partner, son, daughter, and orange cat. She can be found online at www.mindfulfamilies.ca.

PHILIP PASCUZZO is a designer and illustrator who works from his home in upstate New York. His work can be found at www.pepcostudio.com.

It was an ordinary day, full of ordinary things.

After school, Elliot went to his neighbor Carmen's house. He always went there until his parents got home from work.

"Hi Carmen!"

"Hi Elliot! How was school?"

"It was okay.
May I have a snack before
I start my homework?"
asked Elliot.

"Of course.
Would you like an apple?"

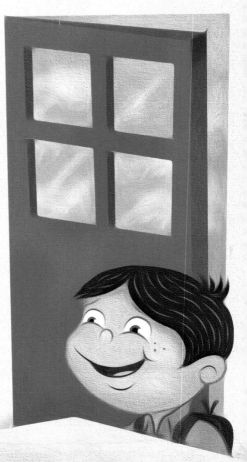

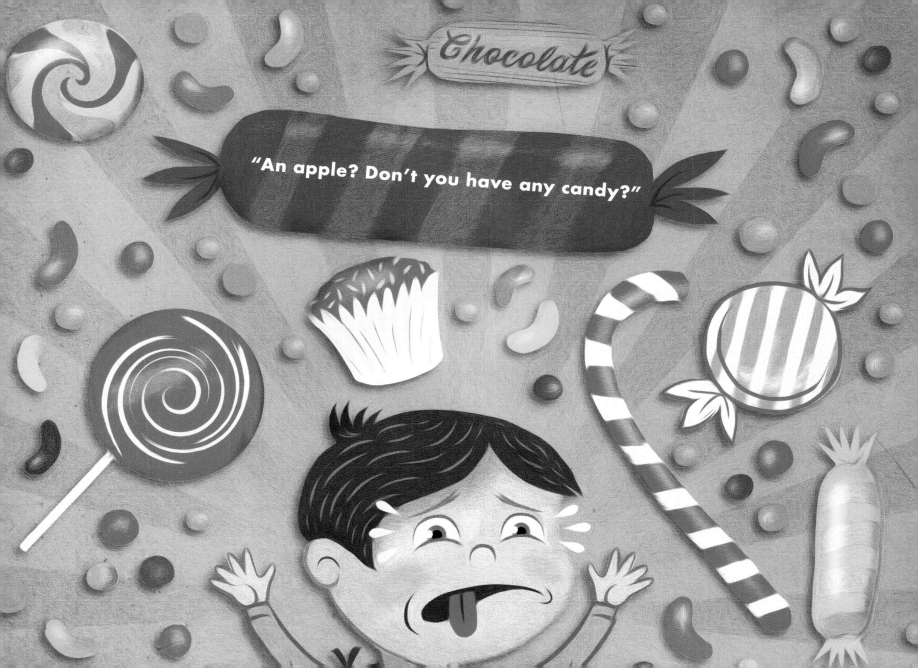

"Sorry, I'm all out of candy.
But try this apple.
It's very special."

"What's so special about it? It looks pretty ordinary to me."

"Oh, this is no ordinary apple," said Carmen.
"It might surprise you."

"Will it give me superpowers?"

"I don't know. Would you like to find out?" she asked.

"How?" said Elliot.

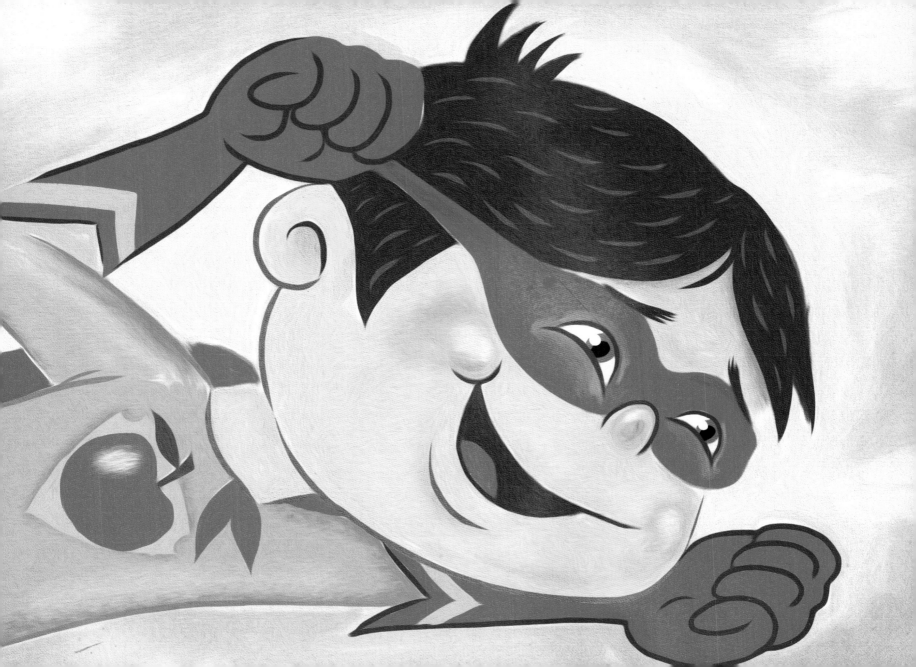

"Eat the apple like you've never had one before. Only then will you discover what makes it so special."

"But I've eaten about a million apples. How can I do that?" asked Elliot.

"First off, tell me this:
What color is the apple?"

"It's red," Elliot said quickly.

"Is it? Look VERY closely."

Elliot rolled the apple around in his hands.
He noticed that some spots were pure red,
some were green, and others were a little
brown. There were even a few dull, black
speckles.

"Hmmm. There are so many different
colors here. I guess it isn't just red!"

"A very good observation. And what does it feel like?"

"Ummm..." Elliot looked puzzled. "Like an apple?" he said.

Carmen laughed. "Slowly feel it with your fingers. What do you notice?"

"It's a little cold... Some parts are smooth, and others are bumpy. Some places are hard, and some are a little soft. Neat!"

Elliot was about to take a bite when Carmen said, "Not yet! You haven't LISTENED to it."

"LISTEN to the apple? How weird!" Elliot thought.

Feeling a little silly,
he held it up to his ear,
expecting to hear
something.

He heard nothing.

"Is that the only way to
listen to an apple?"
Carmen asked.

Elliot got an idea.

He tossed the apple up in the air. As it landed in his hands, he heard a hollow *THWAP*.

Elliot smiled. He'd probably made that sound a million times before but never actually heard it.

"Now do I take a bite?"
he asked, growing impatient.

"Not quite yet.
What does it smell like?"

Elliot took a sniff. "Umm. Fruity, I guess.
And a little like flowers. And springtime."

After another moment he laughed.
"It also feels cool and
smooth against my nose."

Carmen smiled.

"Can I take a bite now?" Elliot could feel his tummy rumbling.

"Sure," said Carmen. "But I wonder what else you might discover if you bite it very, very slowly."

Elliot really wanted to figure out the secret of the apple, so he decided to try. As he held it up to his lips, he noticed his mouth was already watering! He was pretty sure this had never happened with an apple before.

As his teeth sunk in, he heard a loud

crisp

CRUNCH!

He noticed the sweet appley juiciness in his mouth and little juice drops tickling his chin. The peel felt stringy; the flesh felt cool and spongy. Then came a burst of the familiar, fresh appley smell.

"Notice what the apple tastes like in different parts of your mouth. You can do this if you chew it very slowly and roll it around. Oh, and try not to swallow just yet! Do you think you can do that?" asked Carmen.

Elliot nodded. First, he chewed on one side, and then the other. Next, he rolled the chewed-up apple around in his mouth.

He tasted it on the back of his tongue, the center, the front, one side, the other side... He even tried *smooshing* the apple against the top of his mouth.

He really wanted to swallow the whole time but was determined not to; he was going to discover the secret!

"Are you ready to swallow it now?"

"*Yesh pleashe,*" Elliot said, through his apple-filled mouth.

"Go ahead! See what you notice as the apple travels to your belly. It may help if you close your eyes."

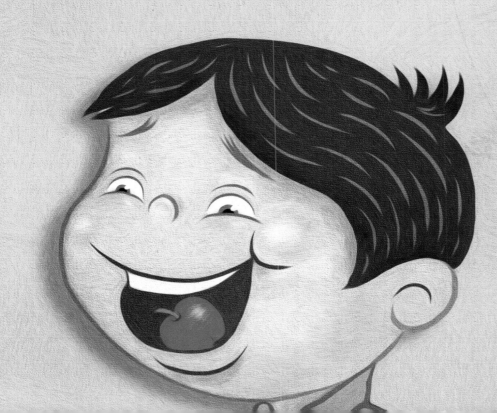

Elliot closed his eyes
and concentrated as
he swallowed. He
could feel the
moistness of the apple
as it went down his
throat. His belly had
stopped rumbling and
even
felt a little more full.

"What did you notice?" asked Carmen.

"You know, the apple DID taste different at the front of my mouth than at the back," Elliot said. "In one part, it was sweet. In another, kind of tart. Like two fruits in one!"

Even after all this time, Elliot still wasn't sure what made this particular apple so special. Yes, it was more colorful, more tasty, more fragrant, and more noisy than any apple he had ever eaten. In fact, it was the most appley apple ever! But why?

"What's the secret?" Elliot asked.
"Why is this apple so super appley?
What did you do to make it that way?"

"Ahh," said Carmen. "It's not what *I* did
that made it so special. It's what YOU
did!"

Elliot looked proud. "What I did?"

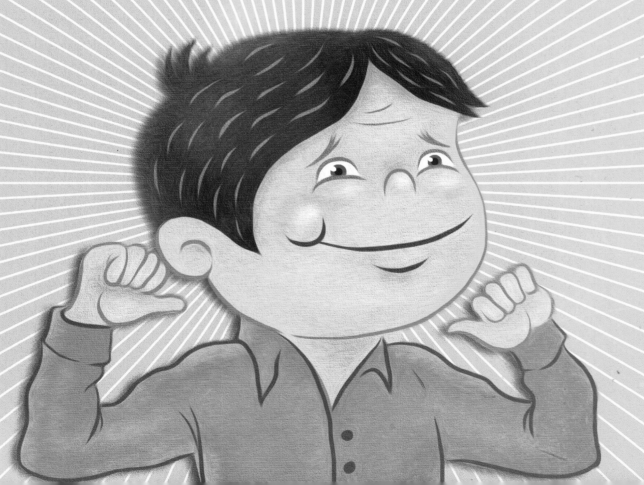

"By slowing down when eating this apple, and being curious about how it looks, feels, sounds, smells, and tastes, YOU made it extraordinary. And you know what? You can do this with any food."

Elliot thought about this for a moment.
His eyes sparkled. "Jelly beans?"

"Sure!"

"Ice cream?"

"Absolutely."

"Even macaroni and cheese?"
Elliot couldn't imagine macaroni and cheese being even better.

"Yes, even macaroni and cheese."

"Wow!"

"You know, Elliot, you can try this with foods that AREN'T your favorite, too."

"Really? I don't know. Broccoli is pretty gross. And peas. I don't think I could ever eat peas so slowly."

"Well, it's worth a try. Maybe start with one little pea. You might be amazed at what you discover, just like with the apple."

Elliot thought for a moment. Then he slowly and mindfully ate the rest of the apple.

He thought about all the foods he could eat this way. He couldn't wait to show his family and friends!

Then a huge smile washed over his face. He remembered that today was Friday...

and that meant...

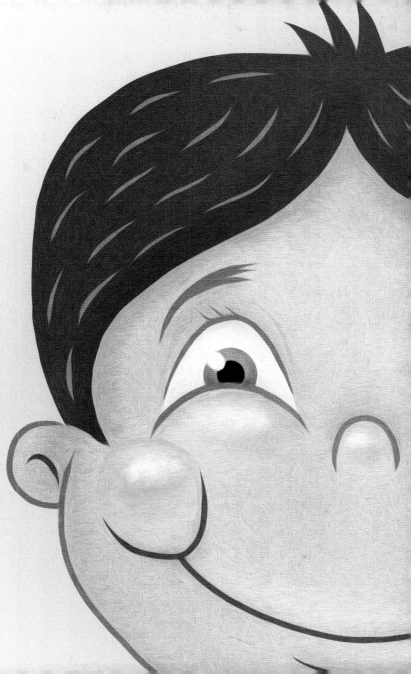

Pizza night!